Laura's Great Guide to Fitness

How to Stay Healthy Throughout the Ages

Laura Gudipalley

authorHOUSE®

AuthorHouse™
1663 Liberty Drive
Bloomington, IN 47403
www.authorhouse.com
Phone: 1 (800) 839-8640

You may contact the writer Laura Gudipalley at
6784723719 for more useful information.

Published by AuthorHouse 09/27/2016

ISBN: 978-1-5246-1851-3 (sc)
ISBN: 978-1-5246-1850-6 (e)

Print information available on the last page.

This book is printed on acid-free paper.

TABLE OF CONTENTS

INTRO

Home Gyms
Exercising at home saves time and money! Having
a gym in the convenience of one's own home is Safe,
Comfortable, Convenient, and did I mention Clean?
Why wait for a sweaty exercise machine, or stand in
line for a spin class, to find that you still need to
fight over a set of slippery dumbbells? I am here to
save the day! Have your personal retreat built to
your own Standards and Specifications and Live
each day to the Fullest!!!
Gym Members
<u>Interior Design and Space Planning</u>
<u>Fitness Products</u>
<u>Personal Fitness Training</u>
<u>Bootcamp in the Park</u>
<u>Electronics</u>
You
Parking Spaces Available!
Exercise is #1 in SAVING YOU $$$

Just think of your Own Home Gym
as a Personal Retreat. Rethink
what your life could be like with
more money and more time!
Money you will save on hospital bills,
medical bills, gym fees, gas,
and expensive trainers who never quite get the job done...
The Possibilities are Endless!
Custom Home Gyms is a full-service,

Interior
Design Firm with a distinguished reputation.
Whether you
Need help with minor updating, large-scale
Renovations or
New construction, I will achieve the look you want.
Always
On time and within budget! When on the move
It is hard to
Find time to go to the gym. This is why I bring the
Gym to you.
This is called "geographical mobility," the ability
To move from
Location to location and still go about your
Daily routines.
This system works! Leave the accountability
To the
Professionals and the looks to the
Interior Designers!

TIPS ON EATING OUT

1) Share an entire entre or take 1/2 home.

2) Order water with Lemon or Lime to Drink instead of other drinks.

3) Order a Salad or Soup with a Side of Protein.

4) Skip the Carbohydrates!

5) 1x a month for an average eater you may go out to a normal restaurant dining experience.

   The rest should be soups and salads.

6) Do not feel like you have to order everything on the menu.

At Home Eating

1) Small Portions: 4-6 oz. of meat, 6-8 oz. of vegetables, no starch or carbohydrates!

2) Try using a grill or a wok with no oil or cook with water or PAM (nonstick), NO Butter!

3) Do not eat until you are full!

4) Try snacking, 4-6 small meals a day, instead of larger meals.

5) Eat your vegetables, proteins, and fruits on your schedule as planned for your daily allowance.

GRABBING A PICKNICK

1) Do not go and buy a pack of KFC Fried Chicken every weekend with french fries.

   Instead try a Fresh Salad or a small sub from a local market with some fruit or some fruit with some cheese and crackers.

2) Remember your H20; when you are picnicking, you do not want to fill up on carbonated drinks.

DRINKING?

1) Drinking is ok in moderation, but every day is not ok!

2) 1-2 glasses of wine or a beer on the weekend is fine, but remember that for every wine or beer it is an extra 120 calories wasted.

3) Drinking can put on a gut to your belly faster than eating donuts every day!

4) Remember your H20! You must drink 32 oz. of water daily, that is roughly 2 full glasses of water every 4 hours.

WHAT IS IN YOUR CHILDS SCHOOL LUNCH? WHAT YOU CAN DO TO INCREASE HIS OR HER VEGETABLES, PROTEINS, AND FRUITS

Since I have a son. Nathan and he is a blessing to me, I wonder what he eats at school every day. I ask him every day when I pick him up from school, "What did you eat for lunch today?" Half the time. he doesn't know, and sometimes he remembers and can tell me exactly what he ate. Lately, we have been working on a plan to get more vegetables, proteins, and fruits in his school lunch. He was so excited when his school added green beans to the menu. It was the first thing he told me when he got into my car when I picked him up that day. It is very important to know what your child is eating on a daily basis. Let your Headmaster know that the students need more of a certain food in thier diet and they will be sure to try to meet your needs.

DAILY EXERCISE

1-2 hours a day for adults 5 days a week

1 hour a day for kids 5 days a week

It is so important to include some type of daily exercise in your daily routine. Whether it is walking, jogging, swimming, vacuuming, or doing sit-ups.

HOME TRAINING

Home Training is important because you cannot always make it to the gym from your home. All exercises done in a major gym can be done in your own home, with the right equipment. You do not need much room and with the correct equipment you will get even more exercise at a home gym then you would at any other gym. You have more focus, you do not need to wait for any machine, you can listen to your own music, you can clean it when you want, and there is no less down time, so your workouts are higher intensity, and you pick which equipment you want. Plus you do not have to go out in the rain and traffic to get there, or pay a toll. You home gym is catored to you. It is what you make of it that is the fun part!

GET OUT DOORS!

Do not forget to get outdoors! It is so important to get outside and exercise as well. Fresh air is so healing for you mind, body, and Go for a walk, run, bike ride, or go swimming. You can stretch or meditate or just relax and read a book! Learn how to clear your mind and suppress your stress.

DON'T FORGET TO SHOP ONLINE AT WWW.CUSTOMGYMSONLINE. COM FOR YOUR FITNESS EQUIPMENT AND HEALTH ADVISE.

Custom Home Gyms, LLC. is your one stop shop to get you fitness ready at www.customgymsonline.com

Custom Home Gyms, LLC.

Get Fit in the Comfort of Your Own Home!

WHY SO MANY DIETS FAIL?

Following a calorie restricted diet will obviously result in weight loss. But what about that Boom-a-rang effect, when you get hungry again? Fad Diets provide you with a structured plan to follow, but at a close up angle, these trendy diets may be deficient in important macro and micro nutrients! Most of these diets do not provide adequate nutrition and therefore are not meant for individuals who are on an athletic training or fitness program.

Sample Meal Plan

Breakfast

Egg and Cheese Burrito with Honeydew Melon

Lunch

Curried Turkey Salad with Walnuts and Flat Bread

Dinner

Foiled Fish with Couscouse and Balsamic Tomatoes

Afternoon Snack

Yogurt with Raspberries and Almonds

Late-Night Snack

Mini Pita Pizza

*Give Menu, Ingredients, and Full Diet list of each menu.

The most important factors in losing weight and maintaining weight include not overeating, eating a low fat diet (less than 25% of you daily calories) with high fiber, moderate protein, and high carbohydrates. Eating whole foods, organic whenever possible, and eating 5 or more smaller meals a day, with regular exercise!

YOU ARE WHAT YOU EAT!

THE GLYCEMIC IMPACT DIET (GI DIET)

A healthy nutrition plan you can easily follow for life. It balances unrefined complex carbohydrates with lean protein and healthy fat to help you stabilize blood sugars and increase energy while losing weight. Feel fuller longer and avoid those nasty sugar "highs" and "lows."

Foods That Are NOT Allowed!

No foods are specifically excluded- you will choose your meals from a wide variety of delicious meals and snacks.

Risks!

The Glycemic Impact Meal Plan is a generally healthy meal plan. If you have additional specific dietary or medical needs, you may with to review your plans with a healthcare provider or nutritionist.

LAURA'S DAILY MENU

Daily Vitamins and Hydrocutmax 2x per day (or other supplement) 7:00 and 12:00 noon

Daily Exercise (1-2 Hours) 8:00 am and 4:00 pm

At least 30-36 oz. Water per Day (2 cups per meal)

> (360 calories per meal 2x a day with 1 meal replacement of 150 calories or less*)

Breakfast: Around 7:00 AM

> 1 Coffee, 1 Egg
>
> 1 Coffee, Cereal (1 cup)
>
> 1 Coffee, Oatmeal (1 cup)
>
> 1 Coffee, Fruit and Yougart (1 cup)
>
> 1 Coffee, 1 Banana
>
> Water 8 oz. or Fat Free Lactaid Milk with 1

scoop of Hydrocut Zero or whey protein powder and 1 scoop L-glutamine powder

8:00 am Exercise

Mid-Morning Snack: 10:00 AM

> 1 Cup Fresh Squeezed Juice
>
> 1 Piece of Fruit
>
> 1 of Breakfast Items
>
> Water 8oz. or Fat Free Lactaid Milk with 1

scoop Hydrocut zero or whey protein powder.

Lunch: 12:00 Noon- Meal Replacement *

Soup (1 cup)

or

Salad (1 small plate)

Either with: (one)

Cottage Cheese (3 oz.) (1/2 cup)

Cracker (4)

Tuna Fish (3 oz.)

Fruit Salad (3 oz.)

Tomato Salad (3 oz.)

Piece of Fruit- banana, apple, pear

Water (8 oz.)

After-Noon Snack: 2:00 pm

Hand-full Almonds

Fat-Free String Cheese (1)

Piece of Fruit

Piece of Vegetable

One Rice Cake

Water (8 oz.)

4:00 pm Exercise

Dinner: 6:30 pm

Fish, Steak, Chicken (6 oz.)

Green Vegetable (6-8 oz.)

No Starch

Water (8 0z.)

1200 CALORIES A DAY!

1200 Calories Per Day is about the lowest a woman should go when losing weight. A total of 1500-1700 is the Max of Calories that a woman should cut off her diet at any time!

Meal Plan 1

Total Calories 1200

Breakfest

1 Cup fruit juice
1/2 cup oatmeal
1 cup low fat yougart
Black coffe or herbal tea

Lunch

Smoothie (1 Cup Berries blended with 1 Cup Skim or 1% Milk and Ice Cubes)

Dinner

5oz Piece of meat or fish, 2 cups of vegetables, small salad with vinegerette dressing, water with lemon
No more than 3-5 small meals a day
Count your fat!
Count your Calories!
Count your Carbs!
Count your Protein!

Roughly 1200 calories a day!
50 calories from fat 4 x a day
100 calories of protein 4 x a day
150 calories of carbohydrates 4 x a day

THE CARBOHYDRATE-LOADING DIET

Carbohydrates are the most efficient fuel for energy production. They can also be stored as glycogen in muscles and the liver, functioning as readily available energy source for prolonged, strenuous exercise. For these reasons, carbohydrates may be the most important nutrient for sports performance.

This Diet has Two Stages:

Depletion-The athlete performs the sport to the point of exhaustion to deplete stored carbohydrates in specific muscles. Then the athlete follows a high-fat, low-carbohydrate diet for three days.

Carbo-Loading- A high carbohydrate diet (400-600 grams of carbohydrate per day) is eaten for three days while training is reduced.

Modified versions of this diet elimite the depletion stage, or require a smaller amount of carbohydrate to be eaten, and appear to produce similarly effective results.

Emphasize whole grains, starchy vegetables, fruits, low fat dairy products!

Some athletes involved in endurance exercise have found that carbohydrate-loaded diets improved their performance.

Sample Diet

Total kcal (2,500-4,080) (2,640-3,980)

Sources of Fats, Proteins, and Carb's

	Phase 1: 4-7 Days	**Phase 2: 1-3 Days (Before the Event)**
Meat, fish, poultry, eggs, cheese	12-18 oz (kcal:900-1,350)	6-8oz. (kcal: 450-600)
Breads and cereals	4 servings (kcal:280)	8-16 servings (kcal: 560-1,120)
Vegetables	2 servings (kcal:50)	4 servings (kcal:100)
Fruits and Juices	2 servings (kcal:80)	4 servings (kcal:160)
Fats and Oils	4-12 tbs (kcal:540-1,620)	2-4 tbs (kcal:270-540)
Milk	2 servings (kcal:300 whole milk)	2 servings (kcal:300)
Desserts	1-2 servings, unsweetened (kcal:400)	2 servings, sweetened (kcal:800)
Beverages	unsweetened, unlimited (kcal:0)	sweetened (kcal:0-360)
Water	8 or more servings (kcal:0)	8 or more servings (kcal:0)

THE 1-2-3 RULE!

Cut back on calories not on daily requirements determined by your daily activity level! 1st Fat, 2nd Carbohydrates, and NEVER Protein!

Rules!

Eat 5 Meals a Day!

Remember the 1-2-3 Rule (approx. 1 part fat, 2 parts protein, and 3 parts carbohydrates)

Example:

You eat 600 calories 5x a day=3000 calories in a full 24 hours.

Of Those 3000 Calories:

100 calories comes from fat

200 calories comes from protein

300 calories comes from carbohydrates

UNDERSTANDING THE ZIG-ZAG APPROACH

When adding lean muscle to your body, this is a great method to use! One must increase their calorie intake every other week while gaining muscle. Your body will adjust itself to the new metabolism while gaining muscle and losing fat weight. You must use supplements in order to replenish your body's immune system! It becomes much easier to get rid of fat permanently by increasing your metabolic rate and not over eating. By increasing both muscle mass and your activity level, you will gain muscle and lose fat at the same time.

MEN'S DAILY MENU

Daily Vitamins

Daily Exercise (1-2 Hours a day, 8:00 am and 4:00 pm)

Water: 2 cups per meal, at least 30-36 oz. a day

(9175 total calories a week, 1310 calories
a day or 439 calories 3 x a day*)

Breakfast: Around 7:00 am

1 Coffee or Tea, 2 eggs, 1 fruit

1 Coffee, Cereal (1 1/2 cup oats), 1/4 cup Fruit

1 Coffee, Oatmeal (1 1/2 cups)

1 Coffee, Fruit and Yogurt (1 1/2 cups)

1 Coffee, 1 Banana

8 oz. of 2% Milk and 1 scoop of protein powder with L-Glutamine

Powder

Exercise: 8:00 am

Mid-Morning Snack: 10:00 am

1 cup Fresh Squeezed Juice

1 Piece of Fruit

1 of Breakfast Items

Water 8 oz.

2 % Milk with 1 scoop of Protein Powder and 1 scoop of L-

Glutamine Powder

Lunch: 12:00 noon - Meal Replacement

        Soup (1 cup)

        or

        Salad (1 small plate)

        either with (one)

        Cottage Cheese (3 oz.) (1/2 cup)

        Piece of Fruit, banana, apple, pear

        3 small Low Sodium Crackers with Peanut Butter

        Tuna Fish (4 oz.)

        Fruit Salad (4 oz)

        Tomatoes Salad (4 oz.)

        Water (8 oz.)

Afternoon Snack: 2:00 pm

        Handful almonds (3 oz.)

        Fat Free String Cheese (1)

        Piece of Fruit

        Vegetable Supplement of a Piece of Vegetable

        One Rice Cake

        Water (8 oz.)

Exercise: 4:00 pm

Dinner: 6:30 pm (small plate)

        Fish, Steak, Chicken (6-8 oz.) plus a Green Vegetable (6-8 oz.)

        No Starch or Carbohydrates!

        Water (8 oz.)

1800-2000 CALORIES A DAY!

<u>No more than 3-5 small meals a Day!</u>

Count Your Fat

Count Your Calories

Count Your Carbohydrates

Count Your Protein

KID'S DAILY MENU

Daily Vitamins

Daily Exercise (1 hour a day)

At least 30-36 oz. of water a day (2 cups per meal)

> (6865 total calories, 980.7 calories a
> day, 326.9 calories 3 x a day*)

Breakest: 7:00 am

> 1 cup skim milk (girls) and 1 cup 2% milk (boys)
>
> 1/2 cup Cereal (non sugared)
>
> 1/4 cup Fruit
>
> or
>
> 1/2 cup Oatmeal or Yogurt with 1/4 Cup Fruit
>
> 8 oz. of Water

Mid-Morning Snack: 10:00 am

> 1 Cup Fresh Squeezed Juice
>
> 1 Piece of Fruit: banana, pear, grapes (1 cup), strawberries, melon
>
> Water, 8 oz.
>
> Mid-Morning snack and Breakfast can be reversed...

Lunch: 12:00 noon (small meal) You do not want your kids to be too tired all day because they ate a huge meal at lunch.

> 1 cup Soup

1 Small Salad Plate

1 Cup Tuna Fish

1 Cup Cottage Cheese with Fruit

Peanut Butter Sandwich with Jelly

Tuna Fish Sandwich

Turkey Sandwich

Afternoon Snack: 2:00 pm

Handful of almonds

Fat free string cheese (1)

Piece of Fruit

Piece of Vegetable: cucumber, tomatoes, sugar snap peas

One Rice Cake

Water, 8 oz.

Exercise: 4:00-6:00 pm

Exercise and Play Time! Ride Bikes, Gym, Run, Walk, Push Ups, Sit

Ups, Swim, etc.

Dinner: 6:30 pm (Small Plate)

Fish, Steak, Chicken (4-6 oz.) plus one green vegetable (6 oz.) and

no starch. You can add a barley or rice on occasion, but not

everyday.

Water or Milk (8 oz.)

<u>900-1000 Calorie Diet A Day!</u>

No more than 3-5 small meals a Day!

Count your Fat!

Count your Calories!

Count your Carbohydrates!

Count your Protein!

Make sure you are drinking your Water
and eating your Vegetables!

DAILY REGIMINE

Meals: Follow 1-2-3 Rule

(Fat/ Protein/Carb)

Ratio

(Nuts/Beans/Whole Grains)

8-10 Servings of Fruits and Vegetables a Day!

Sleep (9:30-6:30am)

Meal 5 (6:30 pm)   **Meal 1** (7:00am)

Workout-ICAA's & LGlutamine (4:00pm)

Homework (3:30 pm)   **Cardio**-ICAA's & LGlutamine (8:00 am)

Meal 4 (2:00pm)   **Meal 2** (10:00am)

Meal 3* (12:00 Noon)-Meal Replacement Low Glycemic (1/2 cup cottage cheese or fruit)

EXERCISE PLAN

A) **Crosstrain**: 4-5 days a week at 130-155+(5-10 minutes each) bike, elliptical, rower, step mill, swim (3-4 minutes of Cardio, a least 2 machines at 1 minute a piece for 30 minutes*)

B) **Intervals:** 1-2 days a week at 6-10 (60-90 intervals hard=160+) and (recover at 140-)

C) **Toning:** No Strength, High Reps/ Low Weight (1-2 Days a Week)

D) **Flexibility:** Stretching and Yoga Everyday

GOALS!!!

Control Your EATING!

Work on Family Obligations

Reduce Stress by Yoga and Meditation

Work on your OWN Business

Stop Drin inking Alcohol

Drink WATER when Thirsty

EAT Fruits and Vegetables when Hungry

Omit Carbohydrates/ FAT/ BEER/ WINE

Exercise DAILY!

10 Bio MARK£RS OF VITAUTY
THAT YOU CAN ALTER

1: Your Muscle Mass

2: Your Strength

3: Your Basal Metabolic Rate (BMR) Biomarker

4: Your Body Fat Percentage Biomarker

5: Your Aerobic Capacity

6: Your Body's Blood-Sugar Tolerance Biomarker

7: Your Cholesterol/HDL Ratio Biomarker

8: Your Blood Pressure

9: Your Bone Density

10: Your Body's Ability to Regulate Its Internal Temperature

Calorie Reduction Should Not Come From Protein, and Should Only Come From Complex Carbohydrates!

Examples of Athletes and Fat Levels for Different Sports

	Men	Women
Runners	5-10%	10-12%
Physique	4-8%	9-12%
Swimming	4-8%	10-15%
Weightlifting	5-10%	10-15%
Wrestling	4-8%	-

5-10 Calories Per Minute Burned with Active Exercise

70%-80% of Max Target Rate to Optomise Fitness Heart Rate and Metabolism

Know Your Metabolism at Rest (Resting Heart Rate)

3 FACTORS TO LOOSE WEIGHT:

1) Eating

2) Metabolism

3) Heartrate

IN (Energy) -Energy Out = Energy Balance

*Do not eat more food then you can burn off!

1 LB. = 3500 Calories!

BODY FAT FORMULA FOR WOMEN

1   Total Body Weight x .732 + 8.987

2   Wrist (at fullest point) / 3.140

3   Waist (at Naval) x .157

4   Hip (at fullest point) x .249

5   Forearm (at fullest point) x .434

Lean Body Mass: Factor 1+2-3-4+5

Total Body Weight- Lean Body Mass

Body Fat Percentage: (Body Fat Weight x 100/ Total Body Weight)

BODY FAT FORMULA FOR MEN

1   Total Body Weight x 1.082 + 94.42
2   Waist x 4.15
3   Lean Body Mass - Factor 1- Factor 2
4   Body Fat Weight: Total Body Weight- Lean
     Body Mass
     Body Fat Percentage: Body Fat Weight x 100/
     Total Body Weight

BODY FAT %

5-7% Men (low)

10-14% Women (low)

1 pound of fat=3,500 Calories

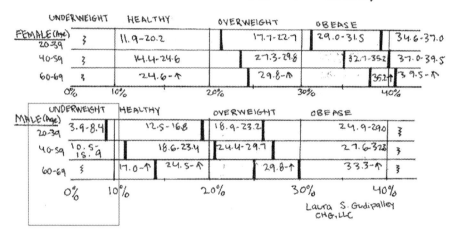

BODY FAT RANGES (STANDARD ADULTS)

Laura S. Gudipalley
CHG, LLC

34

FAT MAINTENANCE

Each gram of fat you replace with a gram of protein or carbohydrates cuts your calories in half.

2400 Calorie Diet: 30% fat (720 Calories) would be reduced to 480 calories (20% fat)

3000 Calorie Diet: (900 calories) would be reduces to 600 calories.

The Ultimate Goal for the Athlete is to keep lipid intake below 30% of the total daily calories! This is to maximize the essential fatty acids and omega 3 fatty acids and to minimize saturated fatty acids and cholesterol.

Siri Formula

Calipers used, skinfold test to
measure body fat percentage)

Adult Women: Density=1.0994921-.0009920
(x3) + .0000023 (x3)2 -.0001392

*note: (x3)= site 2 =site 8 + site 4 (triceps
+ thigh + right oblique fold)

Adult Male: Density= 1.10993800-.0008267
(x2) .00000(x2)-. 0002574 (age)

*note (x2)= site 10 + site 9 + site 8 (chest
fold + center fold + vertical thigh fold)

How to Measure Your Heart rate (Pulse) After Exercise

Your heart rate response to exercise is the best indicator there is to see what your aerobic capacity is. You can find out how fast your heart rate is beating at any given time by measuring your pulse rate.

Step 1: Locate points on your body where an artery can be squeezed against a surface. These are called "pressure points. Your wrist and the side of your temple are the easiest pressure points to find while measuring your pulse.

Step 2: Once you have found your pulse, hold gently against the vein to count your blood flow per second. Stay relaxed and count for one minute how many times you felt your blood pulse.

Example: I counted 25 pulses per minute, that would mean that my heart rate was 25/60 BPM (beats per minute)

This is vital information!! You do not want to have too slow or too fast of a BPM before, during, or after an exercise.

You need to make sure you are getting enough blood oxygen to your organs and you are drinking enough fluids (water).

REST when Needed!

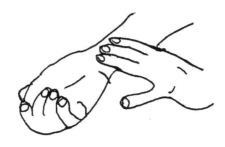

CHG,LLC

10 BIOMARKERS OF VITALITY THAT YOU CAN ALTER

Biomarker 1: Your Muscle Mass
Biomarker 2: Your Strength
Biomarker 3: Your Basal Metabolic Rate (BMR)
Biomarker 4: Your Body Fat Percentage
Biomarker 5: Your Aerobic Capacity
Biomarker 6: Your Body's Blood-Sugar Tolerance
Biomarker 7: Your Cholesterol/HDL Ratio
Biomarker 8: Your Blood Pressure
Biomarker 9: Your Bone Density
Biomarker 10: Your Body's Ability to Regulate Its
                     Internal Temperature

ESTIMATING CALORIE NEEDS

International Calorie (KJ)= calorie x 4.2

Men's BMR (in calories) = 1x Bodyweight
in kilograms x 24 hrs.

Woman's BMR (in calories) = .9 x Bodyweight
in kilograms x 24 (one kg.) = 2.2046 lbs.

HOUR BY HOUR APPROACH: ESTIMATING DAILY CALORIC NEEDS

First you must determine your % of body
fat using one of the mehods described.

Once you know your average BMR for
a 24 hour period, divide by 24.

Add the # of calories your activity level demands.

Determine your lean factor by using the chart
and by using the Energy Expenditure Guide,
to Determine Calories used per hour.

*Remember! Bigger muscles burn fat
calories quicker than smaller ones!

Estimating Your Daily Caloric Requirements

Your Lean Factor		Average Daily Caloric Requirements									
		1.30		1.55		1.45		2.00		2.30	
		M	F	M	F	M	F	M	F	M	F
100	1	1418	1277	1691	1522	1800	1620	2182	1964	2509	2259
	2	1347	1213	1606	1446	1710	1539	2073	1866	2384	2146
	3	1276	1149	1521	1370	1620	1458	1964	1768	2258	2033
	4	1205	1085	1437	1294	1530	1377	1858	1669	2133	1920
110	1	1560	1404	1860	1674	1980	1782	2400	2160	2760	2484
	2	1482	1334	1767	1590	1881	1693	2280	2052	2622	2360
	3	1404	1264	1674	1501	1782	1604	2160	1944	2484	2236
	4	1326	1193	1581	1423	1683	1515	2040	1836	2346	2111
120	1	1701	1531	2029	1826	2160	1944	2618	2356	3010	2709
	2	1616	1454	1928	1735	2052	1847	2487	2238	2860	2574
	3	1531	1378	1826	1643	1944	1750	2356	2120	2709	2438
	4	1446	1301	1725	1552	1836	1652	2225	2003	2559	2303
130	1	1843	1659	2198	1978	2340	2105	2836	2552	3261	2935
	2	1751	1576	2088	1879	2223	2000	2694	2424	3098	2788
	3	1659	1493	1978	1780	2106	1895	2552	2297	2935	2641
	4	1567	1410	1868	1681	1989	1789	2411	2169	2772	2495
140	1	1985	1788	2367	2131	2520	2269	3054	2750	3512	3163
	2	1886	1699	2249	2024	2394	2156	2901	2613	3336	3005
	3	1787	1608	2130	1917	2268	2041	2749	2474	3161	2847
	4	1687	1520	2012	1811	2142	1929	2596	2338	2985	2689
150	1	2127	1915	2536	2283	2699	2430	3272	2946	3763	3388
	2	2021	1819	2409	2169	2564	2309	3108	2799	3575	3219
	3	1914	1724	2282	2055	2429	2187	2945	2651	3387	3049
	4	1808	1628	2156	1941	2294	2066	2781	2504	3199	2880
160	1	2269	2042	2705	2435	2879	2592	3490	3142	4014	3613
	2	2156	1940	2570	2313	2735	2462	3316	2985	3813	3432
	3	2042	1838	2435	2191	2591	2332	3141	2827	3613	3251
	4	1929	1736	2299	2070	2447	2203	2967	2671	3412	3071

WATER INTAKE

Daily Energy Expenditure	Minumum H20 Intake
2000 calorie diet	64-80 oz.
3000 calorie diet	102-118 oz.
4000 calorie diet	138-154 oz.
5000 calorie diet	170-186 oz.
6000 calorie diet	204-220 oz.

7 DAY SAMPLE MEAL PLAN

Day 1

Breakfast

1 slice whole wheat bread, 1 cup fruit, 8 oz. milk

Lunch

1/2 Tuna Wheat Pita Sandwich, 12 grapes, 8 oz. milk (fat free)

Snack

1 Apple or 1 String Cheese

Dinner

Taco Night: 3 oz. turkey meat, 2 soft tacos' with grilled vegetables

Day 2

Breakfast

3/4 cup cereal with 1 cup berries and 8 oz. skim milk

Lunch

Turkey sandwich with lettuce, tomatoes, wheat bread, and 1 cup of sliced cucumbers

Snack

4 oz. orange juice, 1/2 cup berries, 1 cup yogurt

Dinner

Orange Salmon (4 oz.) grilled, 1/2 cup brown rice, 1/2 cup steamed carrots, 1 cup spinich, 8 oz. nonfat milk

Day 3

Breakfast

1 slice of whole wheat toast, 2 teaspoons peanut butter, 1 apple, 8 oz. milk

Lunch

Chicken and veggie wrap, 1 whole wheat wrap tortilla, 2 oz. grilled chicken stips with lettuce and tomatoes, 1 medium apple

Snack

1 cup nonfat yogurt, 1 medium pear or apple

Dinner

Broiled fish (4 oz.) tilapia or cod grilled, 1 cup tossed salad with 6 steam asparagus spears, 1 cup of berries

Day 4

Breakfast

1-4 whole wheat waffle, 2 teaspoon peanut butter, 1 cup berries

Lunch

Roast beef mini sub (3 oz.) lean deli meat on wheat roll, 1 teaspoon of mustard, 1 cup of lettuces, 1 cup tomatoes

Snack

10 dry almonds, 1 piece of fruit

Dinner

Pasta with chicken and vegetables. 3 oz. of grilled chicken with assorted grilled vegetable stir fry

Day 5

Breakfast

4 oz. grapefruit juice, 1 whole wheat English muffin, 1 cup strawberries, 1 cup non fat yogurt

Lunch

1 cup vegetable soup, salmon spinach salad (3oz.) with balsamic vinegarette dressing

Snack

Broccoli, carrot, and celery slices, 1 cup non fat yogurt or cottage cheese

Dinner

Tortilla pizza: 1 whole wheat tortilla with 1/2 cup of marinara sauce, 3 oz. of low fat mozzarella cheese, 1.5 cups of grilled vegetables.

Day 6

Breakfast

8 oz. of fat free milk, 3/4 cup of oatmeal, 1 cup assorted berries, 1 cup green tea

Lunch

Cheese and tomato sandwich, 2, 2 oz. low fat mozzarella slices with 2 large tomato slices toasted on a whole what roll topped with spinach and fresh basil and 2 teaspoons of olive oil and a pinch of salt and pepper.

Snack

1/2 banana, 1 cup non fat milk

Dinner

Chicken teriyaki (4 oz.) grilled, 1 cup salted vegetables, 1.2 cup baked sweet potato

Day 7

Breakfast

4 oz. orange juice, 1 whole egg, plus 2 egg whites, 1 slice of whole wheat toast, 1 cup green decalf tea

Lunch

Black bean salad (1/2 cup), 2 cups assorted greens, 1 wheat tortilla

Snack

4 whole wheat crackers, 1 teaspoon almond butter, 8 oz. fat free milk

Dinner

Pasta with ground turkey and tomato, 1 cup whole wheat pasta, 3 oz. ground turkey, 2 cups broccoli, with olive oil.

LauraA Fitness Plan

Diet	Cardio	Weight Train
4-6 small	3x	2-3x
H20	30 min.	30 min.
Carbs Down	THR	Split Routine
Protein Up		(upper/lower)
5:30:30		Push/Pull/Legs
Food:Cardio:Strength		High Reps/low weight
		High Weight/low reps

Metabolism=Lean Muscle

up metabolism= down fat

up muscle

1 lb.= about 25-50 Calories burned per day

10 lbs.= about 250=500 Calories burned a day at rest

**7 days-10 lbs= 750-3500 calories= about
1 lb. fat loss a week at rest.**

GYM RULES!

No Food

Only Water

No Cell Phones or Androids

All Talk is Directed to the Exercise

Must be Focused and Motivated!

Here to Exercise and Stretch

Become Enlightened

Don't Forget to Cool Down and Stretch

Pick Up all Trash and Throw Away

HAVE FUN!

LAURA'S WORKOUT

Monday, Wednesday, Friday (Morning)

1 Hour Cardio (HIIT)
15 Minutes ABS
25 Minutes Pilates
15 Minutes Yoga/Stretch

(Night)
30 Minutes Cardio (HIIT)
5 Minutes ABS
10 Minutes Stretch

Tuesday
30 Minutes Light Weights
30 Minutes Abs
10 Minutes Stretch

Thursday
1 Hour Bike (HIIT)
30 Minutes Walk
30 Minutes Abs
10 Minutes Stretch

Saturday and Sunday
REST

Core, Strength, and Fat Burn Workout

6 Days a Week

Full Body and Core Plus Cardio (HIIT)

Full Body and Core (Light weight, 2 sets of 30 reps each)

Dead Lift

Squat

Bench Press

Push UP

Pull UP

Pull UP or Chin UP

Dip

Light Sessions and Core

Shoulders, 2 exercises

Biceps, 2 exercises

Triceps, 2 exercises

Pushups

Pullups or Chinups

Dip

Rowing or Biking, 1 mile hard or 30 Minutes (HIIT)

Cable Crunch

Weighted Side Bend

Leg Raise

Deadlift, Squat, and Bench Press Sets (15-30 reps each)

1-Light (5lbs)

2-Medium (10lbs)

3-Heavy (15lbs)

4-Max Weight (25lbs)

5-Medium

6-Light Weight

3 DAY KETTLEBELL WORKOUT

(Full Body)

5 Minute Warmup

5 Minute Cooldown

5 Minute Stretch

Exercise: AMRAP (As many reps as possible)

Leg and Back:

Kettlebell Goblet Squat

Kettlebell Walking Lunge

Kettlebell Deadlift

One Arm Kettlebell Row

One Arm KettleBell Swing

Upperbody:

Pushups

Kettlebell French Press

Single Arm Kettlebell Shoulder

Single Arm Kettlebell Curl

HIIT x 30 Minutes:

30 Seconds High Intensity Work,

2 Minute Low Intensity Work

ex: 60/90/60 or 120/30

HIIT Field Work to include: Burpees, Shuttle Runs, Circuit Training, Swimming, Biking, Power Walking, etc.

Goal: To Build Powerful Core, lean muscle tissue, and to burn body fat.

Remember: You will either hinder or help your body and your training results based on how you fuel yourself.

BEGINNER FEMALE TRAINING PLAN

Cardio: 4 mile walks 2x a week

(Plan for 3x a week Exercise)

Warm Up: 10 Minutes, treadmill walk or bike

Flexiblity: 5 Minutes light stretching

Exercise	Reps	Sets
Safety Squat	15-17	1
Flat Bench Dumbell Press	12-15	1
Lying Leg Curl	10-12	1
Seated Cable Row	12-15	1
Forward Lunge	15 each leg	1
Shoulder Press	12-15	1
Alternate Dumbell Curl	12-15	1
Triceps Cable Press Down	12-15	1
Calf Raise	30	1
Dumbell Press	12-15	1
Side Lunge	15 each	1
Step Up	15 each	1
Assisted Pull Up	12-15	1
Lateral Raise	12-15	1
Leg Curl	10-12	1
Hammer Curl	12-15	1
Triceps Extension	12-15	1
Standing Calf Raise	12-15	1
Back Extension	20-25	1

Reverse Crunch	20-25	1
Oblique Crunch	20-25	1
Straight Crunch	20-25	1
Superman	20-25	1

WOMAN'S INTERMEDIATE FULL BODY TRAINING PLAN

Warm Up: 10 Minutes

Exercise:	Reps:	Sets:	Rest:
1a. Push Press	8-10	4	0
1b. Squat	8-10	4	0
1c. Push UP	8-10	4	0
1d. Dead Lift	8-10	4	0
2. Back Extension	15-20	2	180
3. Alternate Superman	20-25	2	60
4. Plank Hold	15 seconds	3	60
5. Wood Chop	20-25	3	90

CARDIO: 30 Minutes of Interval Training (HIIT)

Flexibility: 15 Minutes of Light Stretching (# 2-3 alternate on Stability Ball)

Woman's Advanced Full Body Training Plan #1

(4 Days a Week)

Warm Up: 10 Minutes of Resistance Training Exercise

Flexibility: 5 Minutes of Stretch

Exercise:	Reps:	Sets:	Rest:
1a. Dumbell Walking Lunge	15-20	4	30
1b. Seated Cable Row	10-12	4	30
1c. Standing Hamstring Curl	10-12	4	30
1d. Pushup	10-12	4	60
2. Incline Reverse Curl	20-25	3	60
3. Decline Oblique Crunch	20-25	3	60

w/ Medicine Ball

Cardio: 30 Minutes (HIIT)

Flexibility: 15 Minutes of Stretching

WOMAN'S ADVANCED FULL BODY TRAINING PLAN #2

(4 Days a Week)

Warmup: 10 Minutes on Machine of Choice (HIIT)

Flexibility: 5 Minutes of Stretching

Resistance Training Exercises:	Reps:	Sets:	Rest:
1a. Pullup	10-12	4	30
1b. Semi-Stiff Legged Deadlift	10-12	4	30
1c. Dip	10-12	4	30
1d. Hammer Curl	10-12	4	60
2. Calf Raise	10-12	4	60
3. Bent Over Lateral Raise	10-12	3	60
4. Four Point Alternate Arm/Leg Raise	10-12	3	60

Cardio: 30 Minutes of Interval Training on Machine of Choice (HIIT)

Flexibility: 15 Minutes of Light Stretching

WOMEN'S AND MEN'S WORKOUT SCHEDULE

Exercise 5 times a week: Saturday and Sunday rest

<u>Monday</u>: Cardio 2 x 30 minute HITT Method

<u>Tuesday</u>: 1 x 30 minute Cardio HITT Method plus Weight Training with Laura

<u>Wednesday</u>: Weight Training with Laura

<u>Thursday</u>: Cardio 2 x 30 Minutes HITT Method

<u>Friday</u>: Weight Training with Laura

<u>Saturday</u>: Rest

<u>Sunday</u>: Rest

WOMEN'S AND MEN'S EXERCISE PLAN (WEIGHTS)

<u>Warm-up:</u>

Walking or Jogging in Place or Jumping Jacks (2-5 minutes)

Pushups (25)

Situps (60)

Squats (60) Front/ Side/ Center 3 times each

Pushups (25)

Situps (60)

Walking or Jogging in Place or Jumping Jacks (2-5 minutes)

<u>Weights:</u> 5-25 lbs. depending on strength.

(2 sets of 25 of each exercise)

<u>Arms:</u>

Front Raises

Side Raises

Back Extensions

Lateral Raises

<u>Legs:</u> holding weights with 1 leg on a bench with heal up

Front Squat

Side Squat

Curtsy Squat

Abs:

Knee Lifts: 100 each side

Pilates Sit UPs: 100

Crunches: 60

*Do Arms, Leg, and Abs Exercise 2-3 times

Cool Down:

March in Place: 1 minute

Pilates Leg Lifts

Pilates Pushups

Pilates Stretches

STEP TEST- STRENGTH BUILDING EXERCISE

Step-Ups or Stool Stepping

Stepping up and down from a stool using only one leg at a time. Do 15 step ups on the same leg, then repeat on the other leg. As you get stronger you can add weight and upper body conditioning.

Do's and Don'ts

Make sure you are in proper alignment with your foot and knee over the stool.

Step Test Scoring

This is a graduated test that forces your heart to work harder during each successive phase. That is why the number of heartbeats you count during each phase gets larger each time. On the following charts you will find your age group and the range of numbers corresponding to your results.

Step Test: Phase 1 Total Heartbeats in Two Minutes

Score	Age 50-59	Age 60-69	Age 70-79
Excellent	102-120	108-125	111-128
Good	121-140	126-145	129-148
Average	141-158	146-162	149-165
Below Average	159-198	163-202	166-205

At the end of the minute, your partner signals you to stop and sit down. You immediately begin counting your pulse for two minutes. Write your pulse down.

Continue to sit until your pulse returns to its resting rate, then immediately embark on phase 2.

Step Test: Phase 2 Total Heartbeats in Two Minutes

Score	Age 50-59	Age 60-69	Age 70-79
Excellent	110-126	115-130	118-133
Good	127-146	131-151	134-154
Average	147-166	152-170	155-173
Below Average	167-206	171-210	174-214

With a partner now clocking the faster speed of 4 ticks every 3 1/2 seconds, you will step up and down off the stool a total of 18 times or 72 steps corresponding to each metronome tick. At the end to the minute, your partner will once again signal you to stop and sit down to check your pulse. Write down your pulse, and rest until your pulse returns to its resting heart rate. Then on to phase 3.

Step Test: Phase 3 Total Heartbeats in Two Minutes

Score	Age 50-59	Age 60-69	Age 70-79
Excellent	114-130	118-134	122-137
Good	131-150	135-154	138-157
Average	151-170	155-174	158-167
Below Average	171-210	175-214	178-217

During the final phase, your partner or metronome, is counting at a very brisk clip of 4 ticks every 2 1/2 seconds, and you are stepping on and off the stool at that pace at about 24 times, in the process taking a total of 96 steps corresponding to each metronome tick. When the minute is up, you sit down and count your pulse for the final 2 minutes and write it down. Sit and rest till your pulse returns to its resting heart rate.

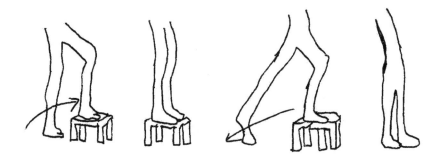

CHG,LLC

KIDS WORKOUT SCHEDULE

Exercise 5 times a week: Saturday and Sunday rest

<u>Monday</u>: 1 hour; Home Exercises

<u>Tuesday</u>: 1 hour: with Laura weight training exercises

<u>Wednesday</u>: 1 hour: Home Exercises

<u>Thursday</u>: 1 hour: with Laura weight training exercises

<u>Friday</u>: 1 hour: home exercises

<u>Saturday</u>: Rest

<u>Sunday</u>: Rest

<u>Home Exercises:</u> Should be done in intervals using the HITT Method, sprint 10 seconds then rest 20 seconds, or sprint 20 seconds and rest 10 seconds for 3-5 minutes. Then start over. You can do this Swimming, Biking, Running, Walking, or any Low Impact Exercise.

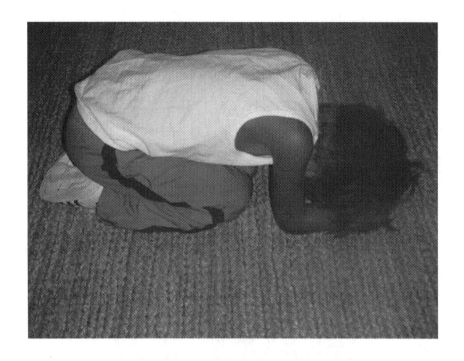

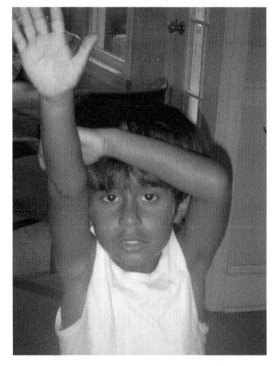

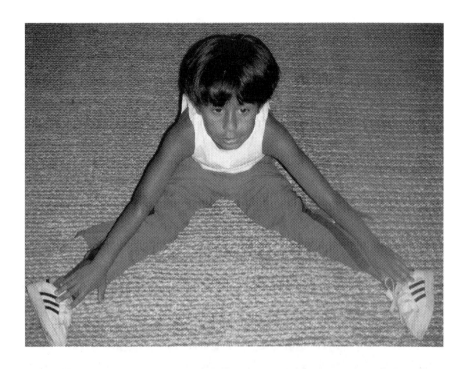

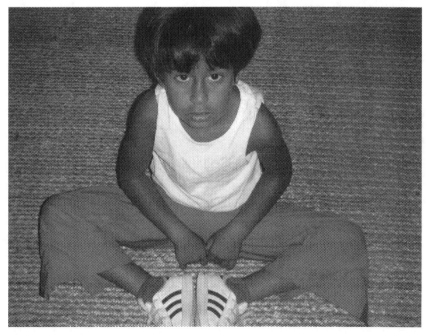

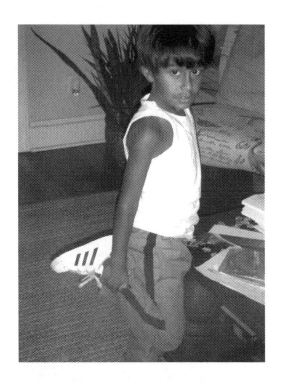

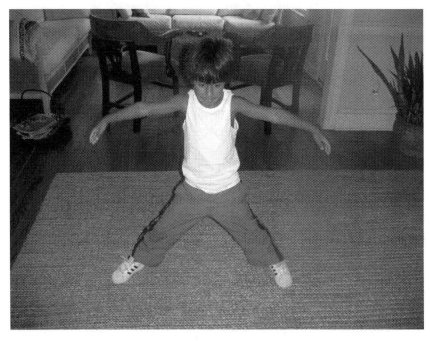

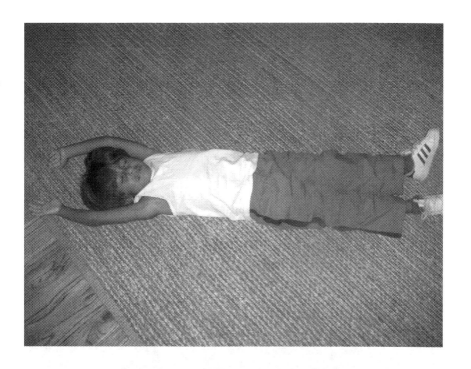

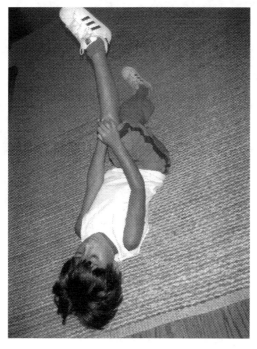

Laura Gudipalley

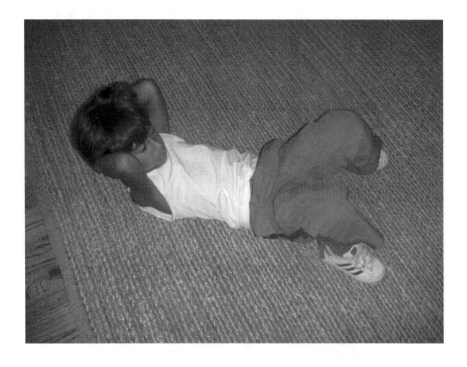

KIDS EXERCISE PLAN

Warmup:

        Jumping Jacks: 2-5 minutes

        Jogging in Place: 2-5 minutes

Sprints: 5 Minutes, HITT Method

Situps: 100

Pushups: 25

Knee UPs: 50 each leg

Light Weights: 3-5 lbs.

Arms: (15-20 each)

        Front Raises

        Side Raises

        Back Extensions

        Lateral Raises

Legs: (15-20 each) with 1 leg up on a bench with heal up

        Front Squat

        Side Squat

        Curtsy Squat

Knee UPs: 50 on each leg

Sit Ups: 100

Sprints: 5 Minutes using the HITT Method

Cool Down: 3-5 Minutes of Jogging in Place or Walking

Mat Exercises: Pilates Sit-ups with Leg Lifts 30-60 each side and Pilates Stretching.

Food Groups

Fruits

Whole Fruits (fresh, frozen, canned, dried} are smart choices. You need 2 cups of fruit a day.1 cup is about the size of a baseball. You can eat almost anytime (Most often) - they are lowest in fat, added sugar, and calories.

Vegetables

You need 21/1 cups of vegetables a day. Dark green and orange vegetables are smart choices. Try to not add butter or oil to your vegetables.

Grains

Try to make at least half your servings whole grain

choices and low in sugar. An ounce of a grain product is

1 slice of bread, 1cup of dry cereal, or Y, cup of cooked rice or pasta. You need about 6 ounces a day.

Milk

Milk products are high in vitamins and minerals. Fat free and low-fat milk and milk products are smart choices. About 3 cups are needed each day;1 cup of milk, 1 cup of yogurt or 1'h ounces of natural cheese count as 1 cup.

Meats & Beans

Eating 51h ounces a day win give you the protein, vitamins and minerals you need. Limit meats with added fat. You can bake or broil your meat or beans.

Starches

Are high in fat and sugar and calories and are not needed for your diet.

1) **Serratus Anterior and Latissimus Stretch:** Reach arm up and over, bending at the elbow. The arm is now positioned behind the head as if stretching the triceps. While bending at the waist laterally, add a slight amount of pressure to the elbow with the opposite hand. Take deep breaths, and relax into the stretch.

2) **Shoulder, Arms, and Latissimus Stretch:** With legs bent under you, reach forward with arms on floor. You can also do this one arm at a time. Stretch the sides, upper back and lower back by slightly moving your hips in either direction.

3) **Hamstring Stretch:** lie in a supine position with one leg bent, foot flat on the floor. Grab the back of the opposite leg just below the knee and pull towards the chest. Keep the stretched leg straight, but not locked at the knee joint.

4) **Elongation Stretch:** This is a great exercise for maintenance of your whole body. Lying on the floor or a mat, stretch your arms over your head and point your toes. Reach as far as possible with both your arms and your feet, elongating the body. Hold for 5 seconds and repeat.

5) **Groin Stretch:** In a sitting position, bring the soles of your feet together. Sit up straight, and gently press knees toward the floor. By leaning forward slightly, you will feel a deep groin, glute, hamstring, and low-back stretch.

6) **Neck and Upper Back Stretch:** lie on your back with both knees bent to alleviate pressure on the low back.

Clasp hands behind head. Gently raise head off the mat and bring your chin to chest. Be extremely careful not to pull too hard on the head and neck. Hold this stretch for 30 seconds.

LAURA'S BIO

Hello!

My Name is

Laura Scott Gudipalley

ASID, FIDER, NASAD, CPR, ISSA, ACE, AFFA

CERTIFIED

I am a Native Georgia Peach! I have had a passion for health, design, and human well-being since a child. In high school at Woodward Academy, at 18 years of age, I decided to begin my career in the fitness industry. I began teaching aerobics at Australian Body works, now LA fitness, and have taught aerobics and personal trained individuals at Gold's Gyms, Concourse, Personal Results, and Alpha Pilates Studios.

I found that fitness was not enough for me at an early age in life because I had such a strong passion for design. I knew that my mission in College was to combine Fitness with Interior Design.

So off to College at the University of Alabama!

ROLL TIDE!

After years of studying and self-reflection, I gained the knowledge of design towards the HUMAN BODY, and grew a strong understanding of my business Custom Home Gyms, LLC.

I now have developed my own company Custom Home Gyms, LLC, offering several services such

as Interior Design Services, Personal Training,
Gym Equipment Sales, and Nutrition Menus.

My clients understand the benefits they receive from each
device they use at home and keep coming back for more!

In order to achieve a healthy heart, brain, and body one
must exercise daily! Less medical bills, Less money
for medications, Reducing stress, Cholesterol, Anxiety,
Depression, as well as strengthening body abnormalities
are all a result from owning your own custom gym.

Why join 2-3 gyms to have the satisfaction of one
gym in the convenience of your own home?

I enjoy showing others what I have learned and
studied throughout the years. In 2008 I judged the
ASID Texas Residential Chapter Awards Entries,
designed several projects, and co-designed the 2007-
2008 Bobby Dodd Institute Corporate Building,
Atlanta, Georgia (Non-Profit Organization).

ALWAYS BE TRUE TO YOURSELF
AND YOUR DREAMS

"Be true to your dream, and keep them alive. Never
let anyone change your mind about what you feel
you can achieve. Always believe in yourself.

Be true to the light that is deep within you. Hold on to
your faith, hope, and joy for life. Keep good thoughts in
your mind and good feelings in your heart. Keep love in
your life, and you will find the love and light in everyone.

Be giving, forgiving, patient, and kind. Have faith
in yourself. Be your own best friend, and listen
to the voice that tells you to be your best self.

Be true to yourself in the paths that you choose. Follow your talents and passions; don't take the roads other say you must follow because they are the most popular. Take the paths where your talents will thrive-the ones that will keep your spirits alive with enthusiasm and everlasting joy.

Most of all, never forget that there is no brighter light than the one within you. Keep on being true to yourself"

-Jacqueline Schiff

DEDICATIONS

I dedicate this book to my son Nathan Rao Gudiapalley.
You are the light of my life my "mini-me" and I want
the best that life has to bring to you. I hope that this
book brings you much useful knowledge of health and
fitness to help you make healthy decisions in life.

With love,

Mom

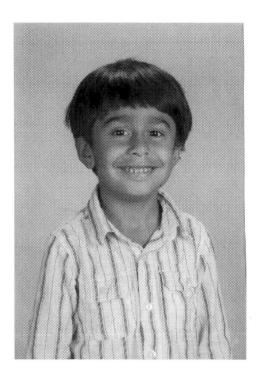

"Time and the Presence of Life"

Time Rewrites itself

Time Repeats itself

Time Changes

Time Stands Still

Time Goes By in a Flash

Time Takes Forever

Time is on Your Side

Time Can Seem Like it is Against You

Time Can Warp Speed into a New Existence

Time Never Dies

Time and the Presence of Life

Tic, Toc, Time is Passing

What are You Going to do With Your Time?

Written By,

Laura Scott Gudipalley

8/26/2016

2:42 PM

On Her Laptop